OXYTOCIN

The Effective Guide How to Induce Labor Smoothly and Effectively Using Oxytocin

Alvaro Dominguez

Table of Contents

Chapter One

Introduction

Oxytocin is a hormone that plays a crucial role in the human body. It is often referred to as the "love hormone" or the "cuddle hormone" due to its role in social bonding, trust, and intimacy. Oxytocin is mainly produced in the hypothalamus, a small but incredibly critical gland in the brain that regulates various bodily functions. The body releases oxytocin in response to different stimuli such as touch, positive social interactions, and even stress. Apart from its natural production in the body, oxytocin is also available in the form of an injection. In this book, we will delve deeper into the uses, benefits, and side effects of oxytocin injections.

Uses of Oxytocin Injection

1. Inducing Labor

One of the most common uses of oxytocin injection is to induce labor. When a woman is nearing her due date, doctors may use oxytocin to stimulate contractions and initiate the labor process. This is because oxytocin plays a vital role in childbirth by signaling the uterus to contract. When injected intravenously, oxytocin can help speed up the labor process, making it more efficient and reducing the risk of complications.

2. Controlling Postpartum Bleeding

After childbirth, many women experience excessive bleeding, which can have severe consequences if not controlled. Oxytocin injections can help reduce postpartum bleeding by stimulating contractions in the uterus, which helps to close off the blood vessels. This function of oxytocin is especially crucial in situations where the woman has a history of excessive bleeding during previous deliveries or has had a cesarean section.

3. Treatment of Incomplete Miscarriage

In some cases, when a woman has a miscarriage, all the tissue from the pregnancy may not be expelled from the body, leading to a condition known as incomplete miscarriage. This can be a painful and emotionally distressing experience. In such cases, doctors may use oxytocin injections to help the uterus to contract and expel any remaining tissue. This reduces the risk of infection and other complications.

4. Managing Placenta Retention

After childbirth, the placenta usually detaches from the uterine wall and is expelled from the body. However, in some cases, the placenta may not detach completely, leading to a condition known as placenta retention. This can be dangerous as it increases the risk of infection and other complications.

Oxytocin injections can help in these situations by stimulating uterine contractions and aiding the expulsion of the placenta.

5. Treatment of Breast Engorgement

Breast engorgement is a condition where the breasts become swollen, hard, and painful, usually due to an increase in milk supply. This can happen in the early days of breastfeeding, and it can be quite uncomfortable for the mother. Oxytocin injections can help in these cases by promoting the release of breast milk. The release of milk also helps to reduce the swelling and discomfort associated with breast engorgement.

6. Stress Reduction

As mentioned earlier, the body releases oxytocin in response to stress. Oxytocin has the ability to reduce the body's cortisol levels, which is known as the stress hormone. Therefore, oxytocin injections can help individuals who are experiencing high levels of stress or anxiety. This can be particularly beneficial in situations such as acute panic attacks or during medical procedures that may cause distress.

7. Autism and Social Anxiety Treatment

Recent studies have shown that oxytocin may play a role in social interactions and behavior. It has been found that individuals with autism and those with social anxiety disorder have lower levels of oxytocin in their bodies. Oxytocin injections have been used as a treatment for these conditions, with some success. It is believed that oxytocin can help improve social skills, empathy, and emotional understanding in individuals with these disorders.

8. Improving Sexual Function

Oxytocin plays a crucial role in intimacy and bonding. Therefore, it is not surprising that it can have a positive impact on sexual function. Research has shown that oxytocin can help improve libido, enhance sexual pleasure, and facilitate orgasms in both men and women. For individuals who struggle with various sexual issues, oxytocin injections may be a helpful treatment option.

9. Postpartum Depression Treatment

Postpartum depression is a type of mood disorder that affects women after childbirth.

It includes symptoms such as feelings of sadness, anxiety, and exhaustion. Oxytocin injections have been used as a treatment for postpartum depression due to its role in social bonding and its ability to reduce anxiety. It has been found that oxytocin can help improve mood and promote feelings of calmness and well-being.

10. Improving Milk Ejection Reflex

The milk ejection reflex, also known as the let-down reflex, is the process by which milk is released from the breast during breastfeeding. Some women may have difficulty with this reflex, leading to inadequate milk production and breastfeeding challenges. Oxytocin injections can help improve the milk ejection reflex, thus aiding in milk production and ensuring the baby receives enough nourishment.

Chapter Two

Benefits of Oxytocin Injection

1. Fast-Acting

Oxytocin injections are typically administered through an intravenous route, which means it gets absorbed and reaches the bloodstream quickly. This makes it a fast-acting treatment option, especially in situations where time is of the essence, such as during labor or excessive bleeding.

2. Efficient Dose

Since oxytocin injections are given directly into the bloodstream, the dose can be accurately measured and delivered. This makes it an efficient and effective treatment option compared to other forms of medication. In addition, the dosage can also be adjusted as needed, depending on the individual's response to the injection.

3. Minimal Side Effects

Oxytocin injections are generally considered safe, with minimal side effects. When administered by a healthcare professional, the risk of adverse reactions is significantly reduced. Moreover, the side effects that do occur are usually mild and temporary, such as headaches, dizziness, and nausea.

4. Multiple Uses

Oxytocin injections have a wide range of uses, making it a versatile treatment option. It can be used during labor, breastfeeding, and in situations of excessive bleeding, making it a crucial tool in the field of obstetrics and gynecology. It is also being studied for potential use in other medical conditions such as autism and social anxiety disorder.

5. Affordable

Compared to other medications, oxytocin

injections are relatively inexpensive, making it accessible to a wider range of individuals. This is especially beneficial in countries where medical costs can be a significant burden on the population.

Chapter Three

Side Effects of Oxytocin Injection

Side effects of oxytocin injection are generally mild and temporary. However, it is essential to be aware of them and seek medical attention if they persist or become severe. Some of the common side effects of oxytocin injection include headaches, dizziness, nausea, and allergic reactions. In rare cases, oxytocin may cause a rapid drop in blood pressure, which can be potentially dangerous. Individuals who have a history of allergic reactions or severe blood pressure fluctuations should inform their healthcare provider before receiving the injection.

Another potential side effect of oxytocin injection is uterine hyperstimulation, which is when the uterus contracts too frequently or with too much force. This can be a serious complication during labor as it can lead to distress in the baby and other birth complications. Careful monitoring and appropriate dosing of oxytocin can prevent this from happening.

Overdose of oxytocin can also cause serious complications, including cardiac arrhythmia, seizures, and coma. Therefore, it should only be administered by a trained healthcare professional and in the correct dosage.

Chapter Four

Conclusion

Oxytocin is an essential hormone in the human body with a wide range of functions. It has various uses, both natural and administered through injections. Oxytocin injections have been used for decades in obstetrics and gynecology to aid in the labor process, control postpartum bleeding, and manage other pregnancy-related complications. However, recent studies have shown that oxytocin may have other therapeutic uses, such as treatment for social anxiety and autism. While oxytocin injections are generally considered safe, it is essential to be aware of their potential side effects and use them only under medical supervision. As researchers continue to explore the role of oxytocin in the human body, we may discover more uses and benefits of this "love hormone".

THE END